T0185625

Atlas of Adolescent Dermatology

Patricia Treadwell • Michael Lee Smith
Julie Prendiville

Editors

Atlas of Adolescent Dermatology

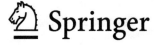 Springer

Editors
Patricia Treadwell
Indiana University School of Medicine
Indianapolis, IN
USA

Michael Lee Smith
Heritage Medical Associates
Nashville, TN
USA

Julie Prendiville
Department of Pediatrics
University of British Columbia
Vancouver, BC
Canada

ISBN 978-3-030-58636-2   ISBN 978-3-030-58634-8   (eBook)
https://doi.org/10.1007/978-3-030-58634-8

This Springer imprint is published by the registered company Springer Nature Switzerland AG
The registered company address is: Gewerbestrasse 11, 6330 Cham, Switzerland

I would like to acknowledge my co-editors, Julie and Mike, for their help. I would not have been able to complete this project without their valuable assistance.
Personally, I would like to thank Erika Faulk for her continuous sage advice on a variety of matters.
Most of all, I would like to thank Eric and William for their unwavering love and support.

Patricia Treadwell

I would like to dedicate my contribution to all the adolescent patients, and their parents, who have taught me so much. I thank Pat and Mike and everyone who has worked on this endeavor to bring it to fruition.

Julie Prendiville

I'd like to thank Pat and Julie for including me in this important project.
Mostly, I'd like to thank Cindy and Kim for their unwavering support and encouragement.

Michael Lee Smith

Preface

This atlas is designed to provide some important information about skin conditions that may be seen in adolescents. Individual patients will often present to the adolescent practitioner's office with dermatologic concerns. During adolescence, body image is a crucial contributor to emotional well-being. The visibility of the skin results in healthy skin being a high priority for many individuals.

The adolescent practitioner will find a number of illustrated skin conditions, a limited discussion of each topic, and useful references. Although not a comprehensive collection, this atlas is meant to address some of the most common skin disorders.

We hope that this text will provide a useful starting point for addressing adolescent skin issues.

Indianapolis, IN, USA   Patricia Treadwell, MD
Vancouver, BC, Canada   Julie Prendiville, MD
Nashville, TN, USA   Michael Lee Smith, MD

Contents

Part VII   Tumors and Nodular Lesions Nodular

Part VIII   Lymphocytic Disorders

Contributors

Julie Prendiville, MD Department of Pediatrics, University of British Columbia, Vancouver, BC, Canada

Michael Lee Smith, MD Heritage Medical Associates, Brentwood, TN, USA

Patricia Treadwell, MD Department of Dermatology, Indiana University School of Medicine, Indianapolis, IN, USA

Part I
Acne and Perioral Dermatitis

Chapter 1
Acne

Patricia Treadwell

1.1 Introduction

Acne vulgaris is a chronic inflammatory dermatosis. The pathophysiology of acne has four main components:

1. Androgen-mediated stimulation of sebaceous gland activity
2. Abnormal keratinization resulting in follicular plugging (comedone formation) in the pilosebaceous unit (PSU)
3. Proliferation of *Cutibacterium acnes* (formerly *Propionobacterium acnes)* in the follicle
4. Inflammation.

1.2 Epidemiology

Acne vulgaris is the most common skin disorder in the United States. Acne can be noted at any age; however, adolescence is by far the most affected age group. Greater than 80% of adolescents have acne vulgaris lesions.

1.3 Clinical Findings

The characteristic lesions of acne are blackheads (open comedones) (Fig. 1.1), whiteheads (closed comedones) (Fig. 1.2), papules, pustules, nodules (Fig. 1.3), and

P. Treadwell (✉)
Department of Dermatology, Indiana University School of Medicine, Indianapolis, IN, USA
e-mail: ptreadwe@iupui.edu

© Springer Nature Switzerland AG 2021
P. Treadwell et al. (eds.), *Atlas of Adolescent Dermatology*,
https://doi.org/10.1007/978-3-030-58634-8_1

Fig. 1.1 Open comedones
of the posterior neck

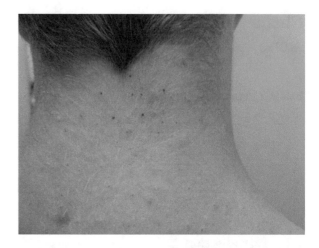

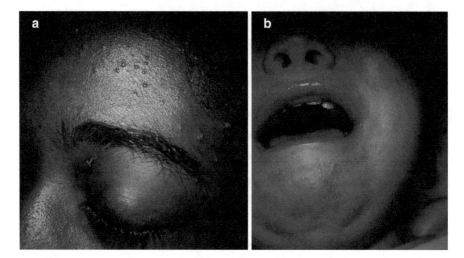

Fig. 1.2 (**a**) and (**b**) Closed comedones of the forehead and chin

cysts. The distribution tends to be in areas of the greatest density of the sebaceous glands which is face, upper back, and chest (Fig. 1.4). A combination of the various lesions may be present in any particular area.

1.4 Laboratory

Diagnosis is most often made based on clinical findings. No laboratory test is pathognomonic.

Fig. 1.3 Acne papules and nodules with some scarring

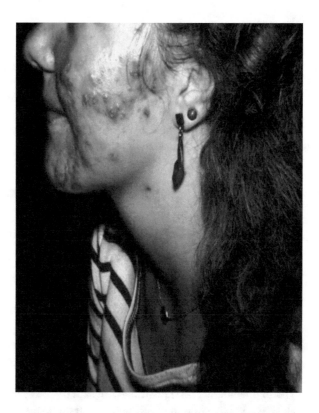

Fig. 1.4 Acne lesions of the back

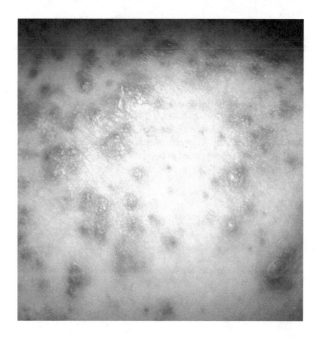

1.5 Treatment

This publication is not conducive for a comprehensive discussion of all available acne treatments. A summary will be provided and the reader is referred to the references below for guidelines for treatment options including algorithms, mechanisms of action, and side effects.

Many patients have already used OTC products when they arrive at the office. Nonprescription recommendations include gentle cleansing, use of non-comedogenic moisturizers and sunscreen, avoiding occlusion, and frequent pillow case changes.

Acne prescription treatment regimens include the following:

- Topical retinoids
- Topical salicylic acid, benzoyl peroxide, topical antibiotics, and dapsone gel
- Systemic antibiotics
- Hormonal therapies
- Oral isotretinoin

1.6 Prognosis

Prompt treatment of acne can minimize long-term scarring. Post inflammatory hyperpigmentation (PIH) (especially in skin of color) is typically bothersome. PIH can be treated in addition to meticulous sun protection.

Suggested Reading

Berry K, Lim J, Zaenglein AL. Acne vulgaris: treatment made easy for the primary care physician. Pediatr Ann. 2020;49:e109–15.

Thiboutot D, Dréno B, Sanders V, Rueda MJ, Gollnick H. Changes in the management of acne: 2009–2019. J Am Acad Dermatol. 2020;82:1268–9.

Zaenglein AL, Pathy AL, Schlosser BJ, Alikhan A, Baldwin HE, Berson DS, et al. Guidelines of care for the management of acne vulgaris. J Am Acad Dermatol. 2016;74:945–73.

Chapter 2
Perioral Dermatitis

Patricia Treadwell

2.1 Introduction

Perioral dermatitis (aka periorificial dermatitis) is an acne-like eruption that can be associated with the use of mid to high potency topical corticosteroids, mask inhalation of steroids for asthma, fluoride- or cinnamon-containing toothpastes, some chewing gums, and physical sunscreens.

2.2 Epidemiology

Although most commonly noted in adolescence and young adult women, it can be diagnosed at any age from early childhood on. Rarely, the dermatitis may evolve into the granulomatous type.

2.3 Clinical Findings

Discrete papules are noted in the perioral/paranasal/periorbital areas which may or may not be erythematous. The clinical findings similar to rosacea with the exception that scale is often present (Figs. 2.1 and 2.2). Occasionally, itching may be present.

P. Treadwell (✉)
Department of Dermatology, Indiana University School of Medicine, Indianapolis, IN, USA
e-mail: ptreadwe@iupui.edu

© Springer Nature Switzerland AG 2021
P. Treadwell et al. (eds.), *Atlas of Adolescent Dermatology*,
https://doi.org/10.1007/978-3-030-58634-8_2

7

Fig. 2.1 Erythematous papules with scale seen in perioral dermatitis

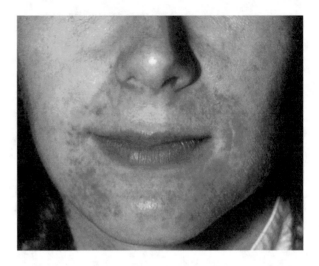

Fig. 2.2 Skin-colored discrete papule with scale in perioral dermatitis

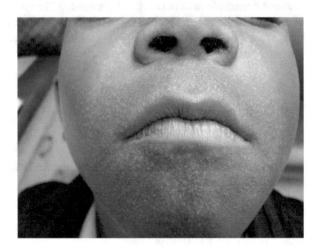

2.4   Laboratory

The diagnosis is most often made from characteristic clinical findings. If a biopsy is performed, histopathology shows perivascular and perifollicular lymphocytic infiltrates. In the granulomatous form, additional findings include giant cells and dermal granulomas.

2.5   Treatment

Avoidance of topical corticosteroids or weaning the potency of any topical cortico-steroid being applied is useful. Treatment options include the following: (1) topical metronidazole, (2) topical and/or systemic antibiotics, or (3) topical calcineurin inhibitors.

In addition, a non-comedogenic moisturizer can be helpful to decrease the amount of visible scale.

2.6   Prognosis

Generally, improvement is more rapid with treatment. However, recurrences may be noted.

Suggested Reading

Ollech A, et al. Topical calcineurin inhibitors for pediatric periorificial dermatitis. J Am Acad Dermatol. 2020; https://doi.org/10.1016/j.jaad.2020.01.064.
Tolaymat L, et al. Perioral dermatitis. StatPearls [Internet]. Treasure Island (FL) StatPearls Publishing. 2020.

Part II
Cutaneous Infections and Infestations

Chapter 3
Meningococcal Infections

Patricia Treadwell

3.1 Introduction

The organism *Neisseria meningitidis* can cause meningitis, septicemia, and/or less commonly pneumonia in adolescents. Of the patients who develop meningococcemia, the majority will have cutaneous manifestations.

3.2 Epidemiology

Adolescents are a group with a higher incidence of risk for *Neisseria meningitides* infections (Red Book 2018). Meningococcal infections are spread through respiratory droplets. Household and other close contacts are affected at much higher rate than other contacts. The length of the incubation is 1–10 days.

3.3 Clinical Findings

Initially, the symptoms may be nonspecific, e.g., fever, headache, malaise, myalgias, and/or cold hands and feet. Some patients may have meningismus, photophobia, and/or vomiting (findings in meningitis). Patients are typically ill-appearing.

Cutaneous manifestations may be morbilliform macules and papules in the beginning, then later petechiae, purpura, vesicles, or pustules are noted. Characteristically, the purpura have jagged edges (Fig. 3.1). Necrotic lesions and ulcers may develop (Fig. 3.2).

P. Treadwell (✉)
Department of Dermatology, Indiana University School of Medicine, Indianapolis, IN, USA
e-mail: ptreadwe@iupui.edu

© Springer Nature Switzerland AG 2021
P. Treadwell et al. (eds.), *Atlas of Adolescent Dermatology*,
https://doi.org/10.1007/978-3-030-58634-8_3

Fig. 3.1 Purpuric lesions with jagged borders

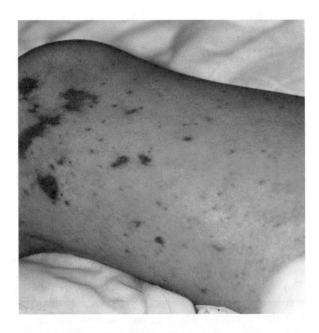

Fig. 3.2 Progression of meningococcal lesions with crusting

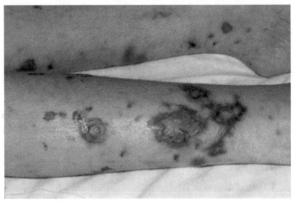

With further progression, patients may develop hypotension, shock, or disseminated intravascular coagulation (DIC). "Purpura fulminans" (Fig. 3.3) is a term used to describe DIC accompanied by necrotic and purpuric plaques.

3.4   Laboratory

Positive blood and/or cerebrospinal fluid cultures can establish the diagnosis. Some public health or research laboratories may have PCR assays.

Fig. 3.3 Purpura
fulminans in a patient with
meningococcemia

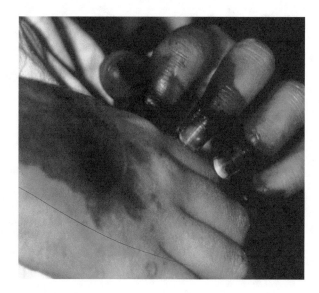

3.5   Treatment

Per the 2018 *Red Book: Report of the Committee on Infectious Diseases* (www.
aapredbook.org) treatment recommendations are as follows:

- Empiric therapy with ceftriaxone or cefotaxime is recommended. Once a micro-
biological diagnosis is established, intravenous penicillin G is recommended at a
dose of 300,000 U/kg per day up to a maximum of 12 million units per day
divided every 4–6 hours for 5–7 days. Cefotaxime, ceftriaxone, and ampicillin
are acceptable alternatives. In a patient with life-threatening anaphylactic penicillin allergy, meropenem or ceftriaxone can be used, recognizing that the rate of
cross-reactivity in penicillin-allergic adults is low. Consultation with a pediatric
infectious disease specialist is recommended.
- Intermediate penicillin resistance is an increasing concern (especially in travel-
ers from areas where penicillin resistance has been reported); as a result, some
recommend using ceftriaxone, cefotaxime, or chloramphenicol until suscepti-
bilities are available.
- A quadrivalent conjugate meningococcal vaccine immunization is now routinely
recommended beginning at age 11 years. It can be used to prevent infection in
high-risk groups from age 2 months to 55 years.
- A meningococcal B vaccine is routinely recommended for ages 16–18 years. For
high-risk groups, individuals should receive the vaccine starting at age
10 years of age.
- In addition, supportive therapy (e.g., vasoactive agents and fluids) may be
necessary.
- Close contacts within 5–7 days prior to onset of illness (e.g., household, child
care, slept or ate in same dwelling) should receive chemoprophylaxis.

3.6   Prognosis

Invasive meningococcemia has a mortality of 8–10%. Morbidities includes limb or digit amputations, skin scarring, neurologic sequelae, and hearing loss.

Suggested Reading

Muzumdar S, Rothe MJ, Grant-Kels JM. The rash with maculopapules and fever in children. Clin Dermatol. 2019;37:119–28.

Red Book: report of the Committee on Infectious Diseases 2018; pp. 550–61. 31st edn. Itasca: Published by the American Academy of Pediatrics; 2018.

Watts PJ, Fazel N, Scherbak D. Meningococcemia masquerading as a nonspecific flu-like syndrome. Case Rep Crit Care. 2018; https://doi.org/10.1155/2018/2097824.

Chapter 4
Herpes Simplex and Herpes Zoster

Patricia Treadwell

4.1 Introduction

The viruses in the herpesvirus group include herpes simplex, varicella-zoster, Epstein Barr, and cytomegalovirus. This chapter addresses both herpes simplex and varicella-zoster viruses. Herpes simplex cutaneous lesions are caused by the herpes simplex virus. Herpes zoster and varicella are caused by the virus varicella-zoster.

4.2 Epidemiology

The lesions of cutaneous herpes simplex virus can occur at any age. Herpetic gingivostomatitis is more common in younger children. Reactivation of the lesions can occur following the initial simplex infection. Genital herpes lesions are generally more common in adolescents and adults than in young children. Herpes zoster is seen at any age, however, is more common in adolescents than young children and most common in adults. An association has been noted between herpes zoster and a diagnosis of asthma [1, 2].

4.3 Clinical Findings

Herpes simplex – Cutaneous lesions consist of grouped vesicular lesions with an erythematous surround. Lesions may be located anywhere, including mucous membranes. When the vesicles rupture, the ulcers are deep seated (occurring at the

P. Treadwell (✉)
Department of Dermatology, Indiana University School of Medicine, Indianapolis, IN, USA
e-mail: ptreadwe@iupui.edu

© Springer Nature Switzerland AG 2021
P. Treadwell et al. (eds.), *Atlas of Adolescent Dermatology*,
https://doi.org/10.1007/978-3-030-58634-8_4

subepidermal level). Crusting can be noted (Fig. 4.1). Some vesicles may become pustular. There may be regional lymphadenopathy noted.

Reactivation of the lesions may be accompanied by a prodrome of burning, itching, or stinging.

Herpes zoster is characterized by lesions similar to those in Herpes Simplex; however, these lesions are arranged in a dermatomal pattern involving usually 1–3 dermatomes (Fig. 4.2). Pain, burning, or itching may occur prior to the onset of visible lesions. Occasionally, systemic viremia may be present.

4.4 Laboratory

Herpes simplex and herpes zoster lesions can be diagnosed by the clinical appearance. If confirmation is needed, the virus can be identified from a specimen retrieved from the base of an intact vesicle. The specimen can be submitted for PCR, fluorescent antibody, or culture (Herpes simplex virus grows more reliably than varicellazoster virus). Both viruses are present in the respective lesions and can be contagious to susceptible individuals.

Fig. 4.1 Herpes simplex of the lips. Ulcers and crusting are noted

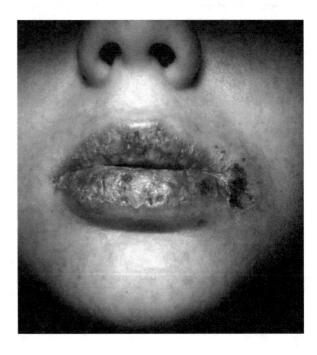

Fig. 4.2 Herpes zoster of
the right chest

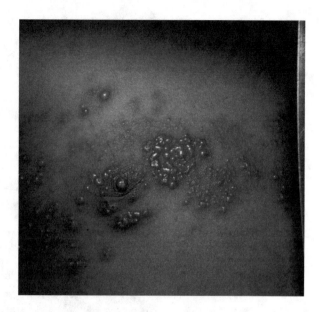

4.5 Treatment

Herpes simplex virus– Cutaneous lesions are acutely treated with analgesics and prevention of secondary bacterial infection. Recurrent lesions can be treated with topical docosonal or topical penciclovir (both used at home as soon as prodrome begins). If recurrent lesions are occurring more often than 4–6 weeks or are occurring in an immunosuppressed patient, consider systemic ant-viral treatment either episodically or on a suppressive basis.

Varicella-zoster lesions can be treated with analgesics and prevention of secondary bacterial infections. If the lesions continue to enlarge and spread even after several days or are occurring in an immunosuppressed patient, systemic anti-virals may be necessary. Post-herpetic neuralgia is less common in children than older adults; thus, systemic steroids are not prescribed as often as with older adults.

4.6 Prognosis

In immunocompetent individuals, recurrent herpes simplex lesions tend to be confined to a specific area. Recognizing triggers (e.g., fever, illness, menses, sun exposure) can be useful – triggers can sometimes be avoided to decrease frequency of

Fig. 4.3 Scarring
following herpes zoster

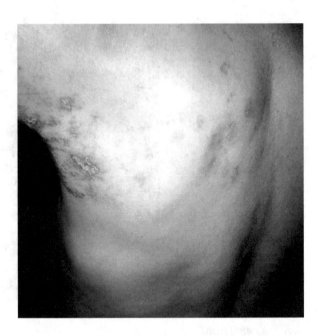

recurrences. In immunocompromised individuals, the lesions can be widespread and cause systemic issues. In addition, any active lesions can be contagious to susceptible individuals.

In adolescents, herpes zoster can sometimes be a signal of an immune issue. Considering this, further work-up should be initiated as indicated. As mentioned above, post-herpetic neuralgia is less common in children and adolescents versus adults. Scarring may be noted (Fig. 4.3). Most typically herpes zoster occurs only once. In addition, any active lesions can be contagious to susceptible individuals.

References

1. Goldman RD. Acyclovir for herpetic gingivostomatitis in children. Can Fam Physician. 2016;62:403–4.
2. Wi C, et al. Risk of herpes zoster in children with asthma. Allergy Asthma Proc. 2015;36:372–8.

Chapter 5
Tinea Infections

Patricia Treadwell

5.1 Introduction

Infections caused by dermatophytes are known as tinea. They are specifically named by the areas in which they are located. In adolescents, some of the most frequent infections are tinea corporis, tinea pedis, and tinea cruris.

5.2 Epidemiology

Tinea corporis can affect any age group. It is most often found on exposed skin, but not exclusively. Typical etiologic organisms are *Trichophyton* species and *Microsporum* species. Tinea pedis (dermatophytes affecting the feet) is seen most commonly in adolescents and adults, and it tends to be uncommon in prepubertal children. Typical etiologic agents are *Trichophyton rubrum, Trichophyton mentagrophytes,* and *Epidermophyton floccosum*. Tinea cruris often has onset in adolescence. The organisms seen most often are *Epidermophyton floccosum, Trichophyton rubrum, and Trichophyton mentagrophytes.*

5.3 Clinical Findings

Tinea corporis: Erythematous circular or annular lesions which have accompanying scale (Fig. 5.1). May be itchy. Less commonly the lesions may become vesicular or pustular (Fig. 5.2).

P. Treadwell (✉)
Department of Dermatology, Indiana University School of Medicine, Indianapolis, IN, USA
e-mail: ptreadwe@iupui.edu

© Springer Nature Switzerland AG 2021
P. Treadwell et al. (eds.), *Atlas of Adolescent Dermatology*,
https://doi.org/10.1007/978-3-030-58634-8_5

Fig. 5.1 Multiple tinea corporis lesions of the right neck and mandibular areas due to contact with and affected kitten

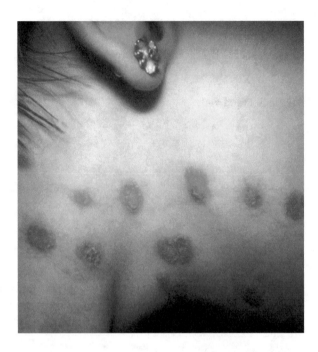

Fig. 5.2 Vesicular tinea corporis lesion of the arm

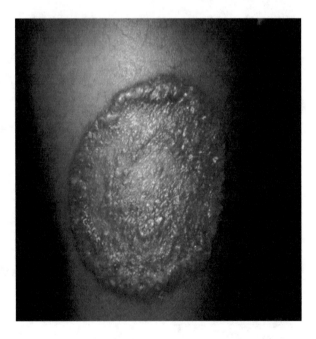

Fig. 5.3 Scaly patch of toe web in tinea pedis

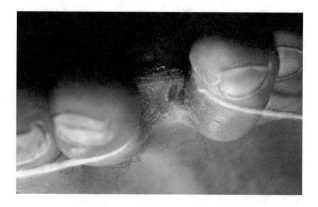

Tinea pedis: Scaly patches of the feet – especially noted in the toe web spaces (Fig. 5.3). May develop vesicles. A secondary bacterial infection may become superimposed.

Tinea cruris: Scaly patches of the inguinal areas. Often itchy.

5.4 Laboratory

The diagnosis is usually made based on the clinical findings. However, a positive potassium hydroxide preparation and/or positive culture can confirm the diagnosis.

5.5 Treatment

Topical antifungals (e.g., terbinafine, clotrimazole, miconazole) are applied bid for 10–14 days. If the lesions are widespread, involve a hair-bearing area, or have significant inflammation, oral medications are prescribed. Griseofulvin – 2–3 week course; Fluconazole – 1–2 week course; Itraconazole – 1–2 week course; Terbinafine – 1–2 week course.

Treating any hyperhidrosis accompanying tinea pedis may be useful as adjunctive therapy.

5.6 Prognosis

Prognosis is good with treatment; however, with tinea corporis, dyspigmentation may occur in skin of color.

Suggested Reading

Alter SJ, et al. Common child and adolescent cutaneous infestations and fungal infections. Curr Probl Pedtaric Adolesc Health Care. 2018;48:3–25.

Chapter 6
Tinea Versicolor

Patricia Treadwell

6.1 Introduction

Tinea versicolor (aka pityriasis versicolor) is a superficial fungal infection caused by *Malassezia* species (formerly *Pityrosporum* species). The yeast forms reside in healthy skin. There has been some speculation that the clinical lesions of tinea versicolor result from the conversion of the yeast forms to the mycelial forms.

6.2 Epidemiology

Tinea versicolor can occur in any age group, but it is primarily seen in adolescents and adults.

An increased incidence is noted in the summer and also in patients with diabetes, pregnancy, and immunosuppression.

6.3 Clinical Findings

The lesions are slightly raised scaly macules and patches which are hypopigmented (Fig. 6.1) and/or hyperpigmented (Fig. 6.2). The most typical locations for tinea versicolor lesions are upper back, chest, neck and/or proximal arms.

P. Treadwell (✉)
Department of Dermatology, Indiana University School of Medicine, Indianapolis, IN, USA
e-mail: ptreadwe@iupui.edu

© Springer Nature Switzerland AG 2021
P. Treadwell et al. (eds.), *Atlas of Adolescent Dermatology*,
https://doi.org/10.1007/978-3-030-58634-8_6

Fig. 6.1 Reddish-brown
fairly flat lesions of the
back with thin scale

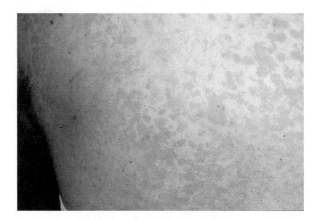

Fig. 6.2 Hyperpigmented
tinea versicolor lesions in
skin of color. Some areas
have become confluent

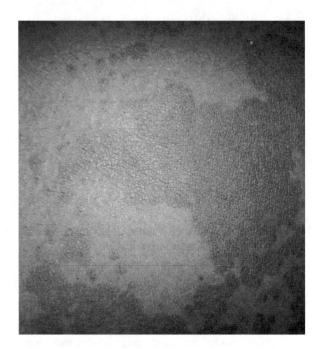

6.4   Laboratory

Diagnosis is most often made with a potassium hydroxide plus India ink preparation
of the scale. Microscopic examination shows spores and short hyphae ("spaghetti
and meatballs"). Wood's light examination can show yellow-orange fluorescence.

6.5   Treatment

A variety of treatment regimens have been recommended for tinea versicolor.

- Topical:

    1. Topical anti-fungal products
    2. Ketoconazole shampoo or selenium sulfide lotion/shampoo
    3. Keratolytics, e.g., benzoyl peroxide

- Oral: varied regimens in literature – see references

    1. Ketoconazole
    2. Fluconazole
    3. Itraconazole

6.6   Prognosis

Recurrences are common and retreatment may be necessary each spring/summer. Occasionally the pigmentary changes will persist despite resolution of the scale following treatment.

Suggested Reading

Brandi N, et al. Tinea versicolor of the neck as a side effect of topical steroids for Alopecia Areata. J Dermatolog Treat. 2019;30:757–9.
Gobbato AA, et al. A randomized double-blind non-inferiority phase II trial comparing Dapaconazole Tosylate 2% cream with Ketoconazole 2% cream in the treatment of *Pityriasis Versicolor*. Expert Opin Investig Drugs. 2015;24:1399–407.

Chapter 7
Lice

Julie Prendiville

7.1 Introduction

Lice infestation in children and adolescents is mainly caused by the head louse (*Pediculus humanus capitis*). The pubic or crab louse (*Phthirus pubis*) is transmitted by sexual contact or by co-sleeping. Infestation with the clothing louse (*P. humanus humanus*) occurs in homeless populations.

7.2 Epidemiology

Head louse infestation (pediculosis capitis) is common in school-aged populations worldwide. All socioeconomic groups are affected. It is spread primarily by head-to-head transmission, and possibly also from fomites. There is an apparent increased prevalence in girls. Head lice may be associated with infection of the scalp by *Staphylococcus aureus* and/or Group A streptococcus.

J. Prendiville (✉)
Department of Pediatrics, University of British Columbia, Vancouver, BC, Canada
e-mail: jprendiville@sidra.org

© Springer Nature Switzerland AG 2021
P. Treadwell et al. (eds.), *Atlas of Adolescent Dermatology*,
https://doi.org/10.1007/978-3-030-58634-8_7

7.3 Clinical Findings

Pruritus is the main symptom but can be absent initially. Head lice may also present
with impetigo of the scalp (Fig. 7.1) and occipital/cervical lymphadenopathy. Eggs,
or nits, are found cemented to the hair shafts, often over the occiput and behind the
ears. Live lice may sometimes be observed. Nits in the pubic or axillary hair, and on
the eyelashes, are an indication of crab lice (Fig. 7.2).

Fig. 7.1 Head lice – with
nits on hairs and excoriations
of the scalp

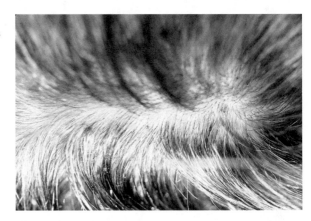

Fig. 7.2 Crab louse
attached to a hair

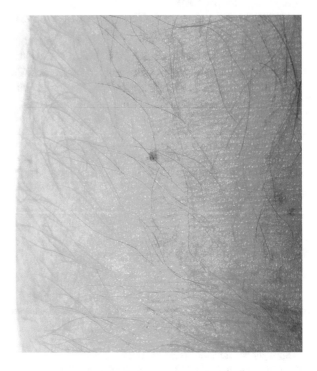

7.4 Laboratory

Lice found in the hair or after combing may be identified by simple magnification, or by light microscopy. Nits can be distinguished from hair casts or "pseudonits" by dermoscopy or light microscopy.

7.5 Treatment

Over-the-counter treatments for head lice include pyrethrin shampoos, 1% permethrin lotion, isopropyl myristate/cyclomethicone, and dimethicone lotion. Topical medications available by prescription are ivermectin 0.5%, benzyl alcohol 5%, spinosad 0.9%, and malathion 0.5%. Nit combing every 2–3 days after treatment is often recommended to prevent or identify reinfestation.

Pubic or crab lice are treated with 1% permethrin or 0.5% ivermectin lotion. Petrolatum may be applied to the eyelashes, if involved.

7.6 Prognosis

Reinfestation may occur due to medication-resistant lice or further exposure.

Suggested Reading

Coates SJ, Thomas C, Chosidow O, et al. Ectoparasites: pediculosis and tungiasis. J Am Acad Dermatol. 2020;82:551–69.

Koch E, Clark JM, Cohen B, et al. Management of head louse infestations in the United States – a literature review. Pediatr Dermatol. 2016;33:466–72.

Chapter 8
Scabies

Julie Prendiville

8.1 Introduction

Scabies is an infestation by the *Sarcoptes scabiei* var. *hominis* mite.

8.2 Epidemiology

Scabies is transmitted by close human physical contact, or sharing of beds. It occurs worldwide and affects all age groups. The pruritic inflammatory eruption is a response to the presence of mites and their products in the skin. Clinical signs and symptoms develop approximately 4 weeks after first contact.

8.3 Clinical Findings

The pathognomonic burrows (Fig. 8.1) are found on the hands, typically the web spaces, volar wrists, feet, axillary folds, and male genitalia. A variable generalized papular, eczematized dermatitis (Fig. 8.2) occurs on the trunk and limbs. Scabies nodules and vesicular lesions are more common in young children. Excoriation can lead to secondary impetigo. Crusted scabies is a rare and highly contagious variant (Fig. 8.3).

J. Prendiville (✉)
Department of Pediatrics, University of British Columbia, Vancouver, BC, Canada
e-mail: jprendiville@sidra.org

© Springer Nature Switzerland AG 2021
P. Treadwell et al. (eds.), *Atlas of Adolescent Dermatology*,
https://doi.org/10.1007/978-3-030-58634-8_8

Fig. 8.1 Linear burrow – pathognomonic for scabies

Fig. 8.2 Dermatitis seen in scabies on the palms

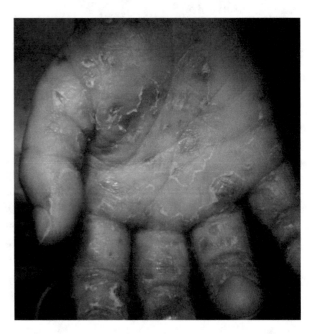

Fig. 8.3 Crusted scabies

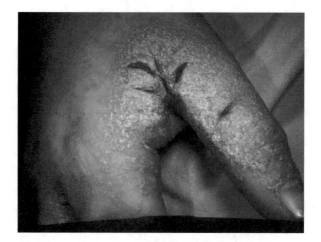

Fig. 8.4 Microscopic
preparation showing mite,
egg, and scybala

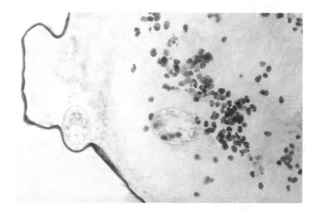

8.4   Laboratory

A diagnosis of scabies is confirmed by microscopic identification of the mite, eggs, or scybala (Fig. 8.4). The mite may be visualized within a burrow by dermoscopy.

8.5   Treatment

Application of a topical scabicide such as permethrin 5% cream or lotion for 10–12 hours and repeated in 1 week. Treatment must cover the entire body, including the neck and behind the ears. All household members and close contacts should be treated concurrently, whether symptomatic or not. Antibiotics may be required for secondary infection. Crusted scabies requires treatment with oral ivermectin in addition to topical therapy.

8.6   Prognosis

The prognosis is good if the patient and all contacts are treated appropriately and concurrently. Skin inflammation may persist for 1–4 weeks and require treatment with a topical steroid. Nodules may sometimes persist for several months.

Suggested Reading

Thomas C, Coates SJ, Engelman D, et al. Ectoparasites: scabies. J Am Acad Dermatol. 2020;82:533–48.

Chapter 9
Rocky Mountain Spotted Fever

Patricia Treadwell

9.1   Introduction

Rocky Mountain spotted fever (RMSF) is a tick-borne illness caused by *Rickettsia rickettsii* (an intracellular gram-negative coccobacillus bacterium). The incubation following the tick bite is 2–14 days.

9.2   Epidemiology

RMSF (despite the name) has been noted in almost every contiguous state of the United States. Most of the cases occur between April and October. This coincides with peaks of ticks and outdoor activities. The species of tick responsible varies by region [1, 2]. Patients or families will often report tick exposure or bites.

9.3   Clinical Findings

Cutaneous findings are common in RMSF. Approximately 90% of affected patients will have an exanthem. The exanthem initially begins as erythematous macules and papules; however, later the lesions become petechial or purpuric. The lesions are initially located on the wrists, palms, ankles, and soles and later spread centrally (Fig. 9.1).

P. Treadwell (✉)
Department of Dermatology, Indiana University School of Medicine, Indianapolis, IN, USA
e-mail: ptreadwe@iupui.edu

© Springer Nature Switzerland AG 2021
P. Treadwell et al. (eds.), *Atlas of Adolescent Dermatology*,
https://doi.org/10.1007/978-3-030-58634-8_9

Fig. 9.1 Erythematous
lesions of the
palm in RMSF

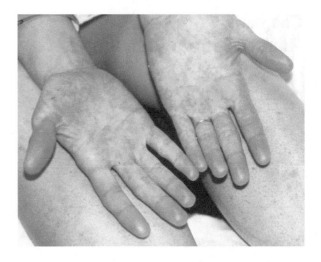

Other findings include fever, severe headache, confusion, nausea and vomiting, and photophobia.

9.4   Laboratory

The gold standard test for diagnosis is the indirect immunofluorescence antibody (IFA) test. IgG and IgM antibodies may increase in 7–10 days after symptoms begin.

9.5   Treatment

Supportive therapy may be needed if the vasculitis is widespread. Doxycycline is the treatment of choice for any age group. The dose is 2.2 mg/kg/dose given bid for 5–7 days. The doxycycline can be given empirically since delayed treatment is associated with increased mortality.

9.6   Prognosis

The mortality rate for RMSF is noted to be 5–10% of patients. Severe RMSF is associated with sequelae – particularly neurologic sequelae, e.g., hearing loss, blindness, movement disorders, and speech disorders.

References

1. Redbook 2018 31st edition: report of the committee on infectious diseases. Rocky Mountain spotted fever. Itasca: Published by American Academy of Pediatrics; 2018. p. 697–700.
2. McFee RB. Tick borne illness-rocky mountain spotted fever. Dis Mon. 2018;64:185–94.

Chapter 10
Cutaneous Larva Migrans

Michael Lee Smith

10.1 Introduction

Cutaneous larva migrans is a common parasitic infestation of the skin caused by percutaneous penetration and migration by dog and cat hookworms.

10.2 Epidemiology

Although ubiquitous in distribution worldwide, warmer tropical and subtropical climates are the most common areas of infestation. Warm moist sandy soil contaminated with eggs and larvae of the animal hookworms are prime locations for infestation. Direct skin contact with the soil allows the larvae to enter the skin.

10.3 Clinical Findings

The typical features include serpiginous erythematous tracks representing the migration route of the larval hookworm. The tracks may be macular or raised and palpable (Fig. 10.1). There is usually intense pruritus, so secondary excoriations are common. The distribution of lesions is dependent upon the area of skin in direct contact with the contaminated soil.

M. L. Smith (✉)
Heritage Medical Associates, Brentwood, TN, USA

© Springer Nature Switzerland AG 2021
P. Treadwell et al. (eds.), *Atlas of Adolescent Dermatology*,
https://doi.org/10.1007/978-3-030-58634-8_10

Fig. 10.1 Serpiginous tracks of the dorsal foot of cutaneous larva migrans

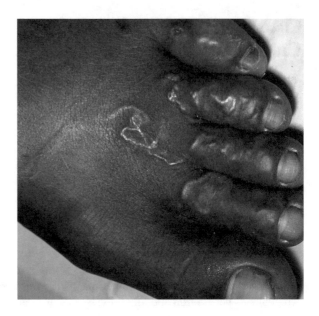

10.4 Treatment

Oral ivermectin or oral albendazole are the treatments of choice. Topical thiabendazole may be effective as well.

10.5 Prognosis

The prognosis for cutaneous larva migrans is generally excellent, since most cases resolve spontaneously in a few weeks. Treatment may speed the resolution as well.

Suggested Reading

Cardoso AEC, et al. Update on parasitic dermatoses. An Bras Dermatol. 2020;95:1–14.

Leung AKC, et al. Cutaneous larva migrans. Recent Pat Inflamm Allergy Drug Discov. 2017;11:2–11.

Part III
Eczematous and Papulosquamous

Chapter 11
Atopic Dermatitis

Julie Prendiville

11.1 Introduction

Atopic dermatitis (AD) (aka eczema) is a common inflammatory skin disorder of variable severity, characterized by pruritus and a chronic, relapsing course. It is associated with other atopic disorders, such as asthma, food allergy, and allergic rhinoconjunctivitis. Moderate to severe AD significantly affects the health, quality of life, and emotional well-being of adolescent patients.

11.2 Epidemiology

Childhood AD may persist or reemerge in adolescence. The prevalence of AD in the 13–17 age group in the United States is estimated to range from 7% to 8.6%, with up to one-third suffering from moderate to severe disease [1]. It affects all ethnic groups.

11.3 Clinical Findings

Atopic dermatitis lesions may be categorized as *acute*, with weeping, inflamed eczema (Fig. 11.1); *chronic*, with lichenification, excoriation, and pigmentary change (Fig. 11.2); or *subacute,* an intermediate appearance. The skin is often dry and may show follicular prominence or, in some cases, features of ichthyosis vulgaris. Mild eczema in adolescents is generally localized, with a predilection for the

J. Prendiville (✉)
Department of Pediatrics, University of British Columbia, Vancouver, BC, Canada
e-mail: jprendiville@sidra.org

© Springer Nature Switzerland AG 2021
P. Treadwell et al. (eds.), *Atlas of Adolescent Dermatology*,
https://doi.org/10.1007/978-3-030-58634-8_11

Fig. 11.1 Inflamed
eczema with weeping and
crusting

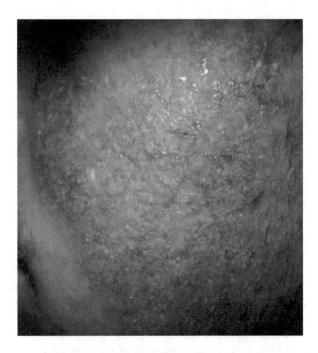

Fig. 11.2 Chronic atopic
dermatitis with
lichenification and
dyspigmentation

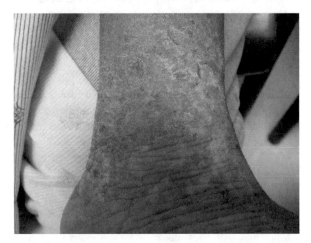

limb flexures and neck (Fig. 11.3). Moderate to severe AD is more extensive with
acute, subacute, and/or chronic eczematous change, and sometimes a nodular morphology called prurigo. Pruritus is the predominant symptom. Pain or severe dis-
comfort occurs with secondary infection. Organisms causing infection in AD are
Staphylococcus aureus (either methicillin-sensitive MSSA or methicillin-resistant
MRSA), *Streptococcus pyogenes*, and *Herpes simplex virus* (Fig. 11.4). Warts and
molluscum papules may also be more prevalent.

Fig. 11.3 Circular eczema lesion with mild erythema and scale

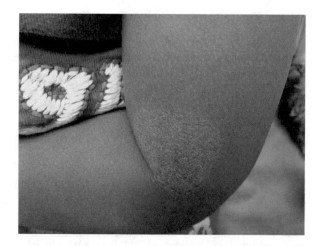

Fig. 11.4 Eczema herpeticum: infection of an area of eczema with herpes simplex virus

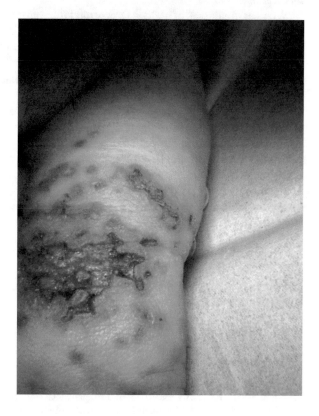

11.4 Laboratory

Atopic diagnosis is a clinical diagnosis. Laboratory investigation may be indicated to investigate comorbidities. Skin cultures and viral studies are needed to identify secondary infections.

11.5 Treatment

Basic treatment of AD consists of avoidance of irritants, hydration of the skin by bathing and application of emollients, and judicious use of topical steroids. Topical calcineurin inhibitors are helpful for chronic dermatitis but are not suitable for acute flares. Secondary infection requires treatment with an antibiotic or antiviral medication.

Whereas treatment of mild AD is straightforward, moderate or severe AD in adolescents can be very challenging to manage. Teenagers are particularly susceptible to developing striae from application of topical steroids. Adherence to a topical treatment regimen may be difficult, and emotional distress and discouragement are common. It is necessary to determine a treatment plan that is safe and acceptable to the patient. Psychosocial support is important.

Oral steroids are only rarely justified as short-term therapy for generalized acute AD flares. Systemic anti-inflammatory agents for severe AD include low-dose weekly methotrexate, cyclosporine or azathioprine. Dupilumab, a human monoclonal antibody targeting the IL-4 receptor alpha subunit, has been shown to significantly improve AD signs and symptoms and quality of life in adolescents with moderate and severe AD [1].

11.6 Prognosis

The prognosis is very variable. Many patients show improvement with time. Others continue to suffer from eczema into adult life.

References

1. Simpson EL, Paller AS, Siegfried EC, Boguniewicz M, Sher L, Gooderhamet MJ, et al. Efficacy and safety of dupilumab in adolescents with uncontrolled moderate to severe atopic dermatitis: a phase 3 randomized clinical trial. JAMA Dermatol. 2020;156(1):44–56.

Suggested Reading

Eichenfield LF, Tom WL, Berger TG, et al. Guidelines of care for the management of atopic dermatitis section 2: management and treatment of atopic dermatitis with topical therapies. J Am Acad Dermatol. 2014;71(1):116–32.

Eichenfield LF, Tom WL, Chamlin SL, et al. Guidelines of care for the management of atopic dermatitis section 1: diagnosis and assessment of atopic dermatitis. J Am Acad Dermatol. 2014;70(2):338–51.

Chapter 12
Allergic Contact Dermatitis

Patricia Treadwell

12.1   Introduction

The most common allergic contact dermatitis (ACD) seen in adolescents is due to plants most commonly known as poison oak, poison ivy, or poison sumac. These plants are from the *Toxicodendron* species, and the lesions themselves are termed *Rhus* dermatitis. In this chapter, we also discuss nickel allergic contact dermatitis (Ni-ACD) based on its frequency. ACD is most often a delayed type IV hypersensitivity reaction.

12.2   Epidemiology

ACD can be seen ubiquitously. An individual comes in contact with an allergen, develops a hypersensitivity reaction, and subsequently, future exposure results in ACD.

It has been theorized that an increase in piercings has increased the occurrences of Ni-ACD. Nickel was named the "Contact Allergen of the Year" in 2008 by the American Contact Dermatitis Society. Nickel is found in jewelry, snaps, belt buckles, coins, pencils, paper clips, glasses frames, keys, and cell phones. Manufacturers in the United States have been encouraged to use only those products that adhere to the European Union guidelines for acceptable nickel release rates in order to combat the rising rates of nickel sensitization.

P. Treadwell (✉)
Department of Dermatology, Indiana University School of Medicine, Indianapolis, IN, USA
e-mail: ptreadwe@iupui.edu

© Springer Nature Switzerland AG 2021
P. Treadwell et al. (eds.), *Atlas of Adolescent Dermatology*,
https://doi.org/10.1007/978-3-030-58634-8_12

12.3   Clinical Findings

Rhus dermatitis lesions are most often noted in exposed areas. The patients will often present with a history of exposure and are noted to have erythematous (sometimes linear or patterned) papulovesicular lesions (Fig. 12.1). The lesions tend to be itchy.

Ni-ACD will be noted in specific area of exposure to nickel. The lesions are plaque like, however will sometimes develop crusting. Common areas are earlobes (Fig. 12.2), posterior neck, and the lower abdomen (Figs. 12.3 and 12.4). Widespread "id" reaction may be noted (Fig. 12.5).

12.4   Laboratory

Nickel content can be tested using dimethylglyoxime. Patch testing can help distinguish Ni-ACD from other allergens.

12.5   Treatment

Treatment consists of avoidance of the offending allergen. *Rhus* dermatitis can be minimized by using clothing to cover the skin and cleansing skin as soon as possible after exposure has occurred.

Topical or systemic corticosteroids are useful for calming inflammation.

Fig. 12.1 *Rhus* dermatitis with linear lesions

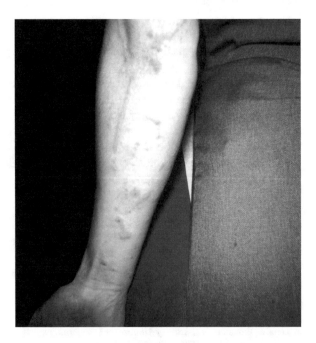

Fig. 12.2 Earlobe dermatitis from nickel exposure associated with piercing

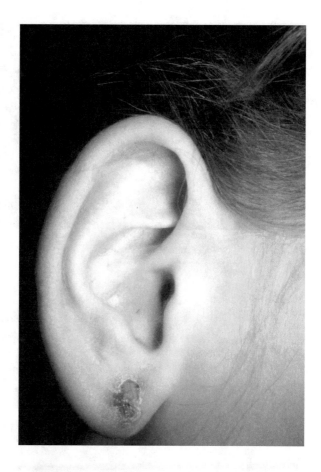

Fig. 12.3 Ni-ACD of lower abdomen from belt buckle

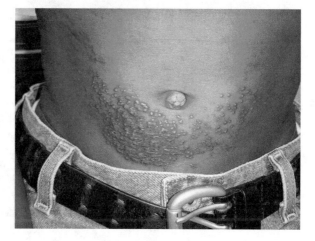

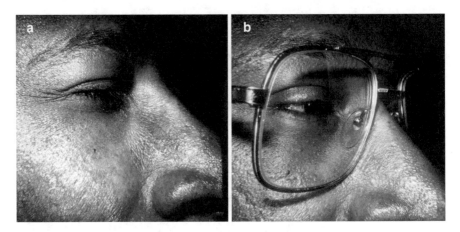

Fig. 12.4 (**a**, **b**) Ni-ACD from glasses

Fig. 12.5 Id reaction associated with Ni-ACD on abdomen

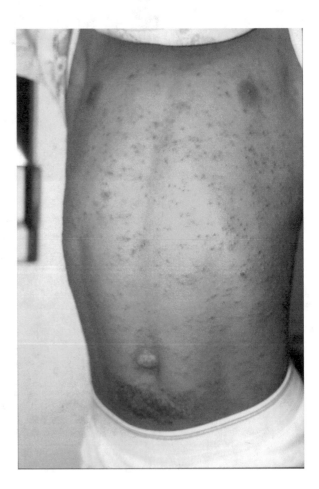

12.6 Prognosis

The sensitization tends to be persistent and hence patients should attempt allergen avoidance.

Suggested Reading

Schmidlin K, et al. A hands-on approach to contact dermatitis and patch testing. J Allergy Clin Immunol Pract. 2020. pii: S2213-2198(20)30158-6
Zafrir Y, et al. Patch testing in Israeli children with suspected allergic contact dermatitis: a retrospective study and literature review. Pediatric Dermatol. 2018;35:76–86.

Chapter 13
Seborrheic Dermatitis

Patricia Treadwell

13.1 Introduction

Seborrheic dermatitis is an irritant dermatitis which affects approximately 3% of the population. The sebaceous gland secretions are altered by *Malassezia* (previously *Pityrosporum*) species (part of the normal flora) and an irritant dermatitis develops.

13.2 Epidemiology

This chapter focuses on the adolescent and adult populations (not the infantile type). The dermatitis tends to be more widespread in the setting of immunosuppression and underlying neurologic diseases.

13.3 Clinical Findings

Seborrheic dermatitis tends to be noted in areas with more concentrated sebaceous glands including the paranasal and glabellar areas, the eyebrows, and the scalp. Seborrheic dermatitis is characterized by lesions with erythema and yellowish scale – which has been described as "potato chip" scale on an oily background (Fig. 13.1). Itching may be present. Scalp involvement in seborrheic dermatitis consists of diffuse whitish scale (Fig. 13.2).

P. Treadwell (✉)
Department of Dermatology, Indiana University School of Medicine, Indianapolis, IN, USA
e-mail: ptreadwe@iupui.edu

© Springer Nature Switzerland AG 2021
P. Treadwell et al. (eds.), *Atlas of Adolescent Dermatology*,
https://doi.org/10.1007/978-3-030-58634-8_13

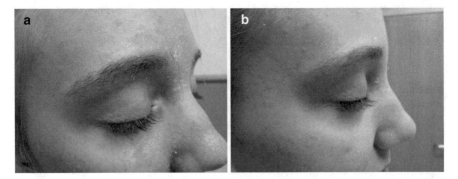

Fig. 13.1 (**a**) Seborrheic dermatitis in an adolescent with erythema and scale. (**b**) Seborrheic dermatitis shows significant improvement with ketoconazole cream for 2 weeks

Fig. 13.2 Whitish scale of the retroauricular area and scalp from seborrheic dermatitis

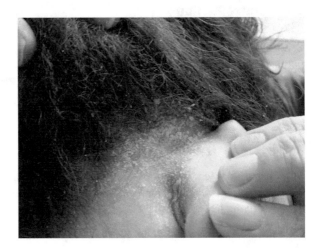

13.4   Laboratory

The diagnosis is most often made based on the clinical findings.

13.5   Treatment

Topical antifungal creams such as ketoconazole and shampoos have been noted to be effective in seborrheic dermatitis (*see* Fig 13.1b). Topical corticosteroids or topical calcineurin inhibitors can be a useful adjunct when inflammation is moderate to severe. Although selenium sulfide and zinc pyrithione shampoos have been prescribed for many years, limited evidence exists for their efficacy.

13.6   Prognosis

Seborrheic dermatitis is fairly persistent, but flares can be prevented with continued use of medications.

Suggested Reading

Baumert C, et al. Topical medications for seborrheic dermatitis. Am Fam Physician. 2017;95:329.
Clark GW, et al. Diagnosis and treatment of Seborrheic dermatitis. Am Fam Physician. 2015;91:185–90.

Chapter 14
Pityriasis Rosea

Patricia Treadwell

14.1 Introduction

Pityriasis rosea (PR) is a benign papulosquamous disorder that can be seen in adolescents.

14.2 Epidemiology

The most common age group affected are 13–36-year-old individuals. There has been speculation that PR is associated with a viral illness. There is a seasonal variation in number of cases and human herpes virus (HHV) 6, 7, and 8 have been isolated in small studies of patients with PR [1, 2].

14.3 Clinical Findings

The initial lesion in 88% of patients is termed a "herald patch." The "herald patch" is most often an erythematous somewhat raised lesion with overlying scale. The "herald patch" typically measures 2–5 cm in diameter and can occur anywhere on the body. After 10–14 days, multiple smaller (5–10 mm), oval-shaped lesions are noted primarily on the trunk and proximal extremities oriented parallel to Langer lines (Fig. 14.1). In skin of color, the lesions may be more papular and/or crusted. The lesions are usually present for 6–8 weeks.

P. Treadwell (✉)
Department of Dermatology, Indiana University School of Medicine, Indianapolis, IN, USA
e-mail: ptreadwe@iupui.edu

© Springer Nature Switzerland AG 2021
P. Treadwell et al. (eds.), *Atlas of Adolescent Dermatology*,
https://doi.org/10.1007/978-3-030-58634-8_14

Fig. 14.1 Pityriasis rosea lesions with erythema and scale, the lesions (especially on the flank) follow Langer lines

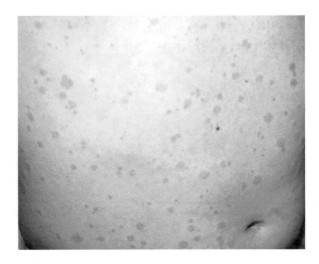

14.4 Laboratory

No laboratory testing is diagnostic. Serologic tests for syphilis are recommended if suspected by medical history and/or if lesions are noted on the palms and soles.

14.5 Treatment

Since the disorder resolves on its own, treatment is often not necessary. Topical or systemic anti-pruritics may be prescribed if the itching is significant.

14.6 Prognosis

As mentioned above, the disorder resolves spontaneously. In skin of color, post inflammatory dyspigmentation can be seen.

References

1. Drago F, et al. Pityriasis Rosea and Pityriasis Rosea-like eruptions: how to distinguish them? JAAD Case Rep. 2018;4:800–1.
2. Schadt C. Pityriasis Rosea. JAMA Dermatol. 2018;154:1496.

Part IV
Autoimmune and Rheumatologic

Chapter 15
Systemic Lupus Erythematosus

Patricia Treadwell

15.1 Introduction

Systemic lupus erythematosus (SLE) is a chronic inflammatory condition that can affect various organ systems. The version of this disorder, which occurs in childhood, is labeled as childhood-onset systemic lupus erythematous (cSLE).

15.2 Epidemiology

Childhood-onset SLE (cSLE) has its peak incidence in early adolescence. The average age of presentation of cSLE is 12–14 years. M:F ratio is 1:5 prior to puberty. Following puberty, the ratio is 1:9. Although no registry exists, estimates of the incidence are typically quoted as 3.3–8.8 per 100,000 individuals. It has been noted that cSLE affects children of Black, Hispanic, and Asian ancestry more often, and they have a worse prognosis.

15.3 Clinical Findings

The most common cutaneous findings are photosensitivity, malar erythema (Fig. 15.1), discoid LE lesions (Fig. 15.2), nail fold telangiectasias (Fig. 15.3), and oral ulcers. Subacute cutaneous lupus is characterized by scaly erythematous lesions in sun-exposed area such as the back (Fig. 15.4). Other findings include alopecia,

P. Treadwell (✉)

Department of Dermatology, Indiana University School of Medicine, Indianapolis, IN, USA

e-mail: ptreadwe@iupui.edu

© Springer Nature Switzerland AG 2021

P. Treadwell et al. (eds.), *Atlas of Adolescent Dermatology*,

https://doi.org/10.1007/978-3-030-58634-8_15

Fig. 15.1 SLE 3 Erythema of the malar areas and nose

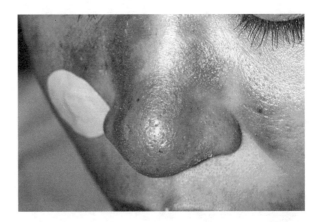

Fig. 15.2 DLE 1 Somewhat annular lesion with scale, hypopigmentation, and atrophy

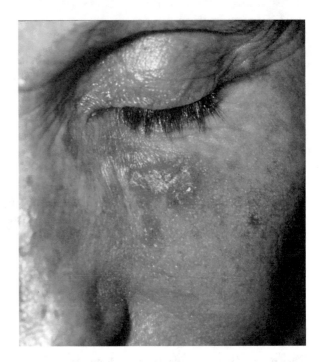

livedo reticularis, Raynaud phenomenon, and panniculitis. Extracutaneous features include fever, arthralgias, arthritis, fatigue, and CNS involvement.

15.4 Laboratory

In 99% of children with cSLE, the antinuclear antibody (ANA) is positive. If the titer is greater than 1:1280 or higher, cSLE is a likely diagnosis.

Fig. 15.3 Cuticles show dilated capillaries

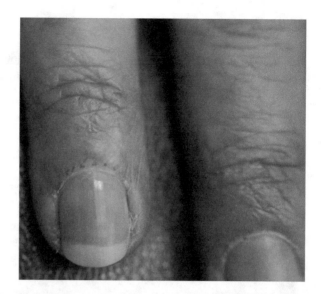

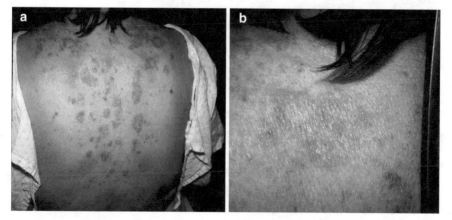

Fig. 15.4 (**a**) Scle Erythematous scaly patches of the back. (**b**) Scle2 Scaly patch in close up

The anti-dsDNA antibodies can be used to monitor disease activity. The anti-dsDNA and cardiolipin antibodies are more frequent in cSLE as compared to aSLE (adult-onset SLE); however, a positive rheumatoid factor is less common.

Urinalysis is an important tool to evaluate any renal involvement that may develop.

15.5 Treatment

Treatment options for cSLE include oral hydroxychloroquine, glucocorticosteroids, and other immunosuppressants, including biologics. The cutaneous lesions may be treated with topical or intralesional steroids or with topical calcineurin inhibitors.

15.6   Prognosis

Adolescents with cSLE have a good prognosis when there is no renal involvement. Those adolescents with renal involvement require more aggressive therapies and close follow-up.

Suggested Reading

Borgia RE, Silverman ED. Childhood-onset systemic lupus erythematosus: an update. Curr Opin Rheumatol. 2015;27:483–92.
Couture J, Silverman ED. Update on the pathogenesis and treatment of childhood-onset systemic lupus erythematosus. Curr Opin Rheumatol. 2016;28:488–96.
Thakral A, Klein-Gitelman MS. An update on treatment and management of pediatric systemic lupus erythematosus. Rheumatol Ther. 2016;3:209–19.

Chapter 16
Juvenile Dermatomyositis

Patricia Treadwell

16.1   Introduction

Juvenile dermatomyositis (JDMS) is a rare inflammatory disorder affecting skin and muscle.

16.2   Epidemiology

JDMS can begin in adolescence; however, peak incidence is 5–10 years of age occurring 2–4 cases per million children each year. The male to female ratio is 1:2–5.

16.3   Clinical Findings

Clinical findings show characteristic violaceous discoloration of the eyelids (heliotrope) (Fig. 16.1), erythematous scaly papules of the dorsal hands overlying the MCP and PIP joints (Gottron's papules) (Fig. 16.2), and other parts of the body (Fig. 16.3). In some cases, calcinosis may develop. Capillary dilatation is noted in the periungual areas with some capillary dropout. Symmetrical proximal muscle weakness is also noted. Parents may report photosensitivity and/or worsening of the cutaneous findings with sun exposure.

P. Treadwell (✉)
Department of Dermatology, Indiana University School of Medicine, Indianapolis, IN, USA
e-mail: ptreadwe@iupui.edu

© Springer Nature Switzerland AG 2021
P. Treadwell et al. (eds.), *Atlas of Adolescent Dermatology*,
https://doi.org/10.1007/978-3-030-58634-8_16

Fig. 16.1 Heliotrope: violaceous discoloration of the upper eyelid

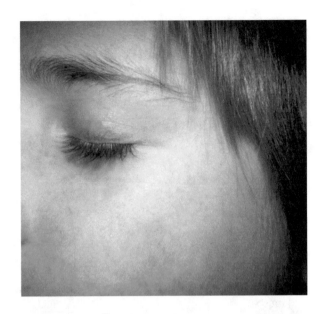

Fig. 16.2 Gottron's papules noted on the dorsal hands overlying the joints

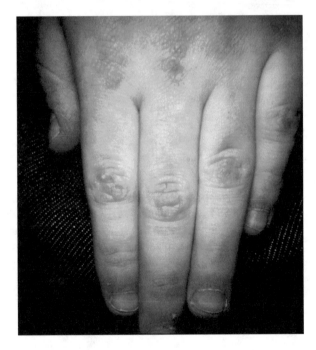

Fig. 16.3 JDMS
calcinosis of the elbows

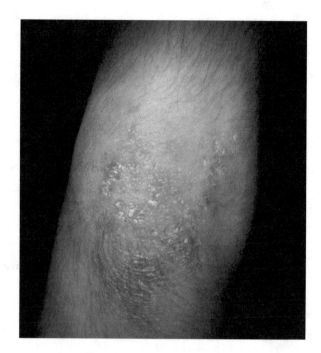

16.4   Laboratory

Laboratory evaluation shows elevated muscle enzymes (serum aldolase, AST, CPK, and LDH). Skin biopsies are nonspecific with perivascular inflammation.

MRI has been used for diagnosis and for monitoring disease activity. The T2, fc-T2 (fat corrected T2), and FF (fat fraction) measurements are helpful in JDMS to distinguish those MRI findings that may also be seen in other myopathies. EMG and muscle biopsy are less often used because of the invasiveness. Muscle biopsies when they are performed can be guided by MRI – since the muscle involvement can be unevenly distributed.

16.5   Treatment

The medications used most often for JDMS are glucocorticosteroids, methotrexate, cyclosporin A, and IVIG. Other immunosuppressive agents have also been used in more refractory cases. Biologics have occasionally been used. Sun protection and physical therapy are also recommended.

16.6 Prognosis

The mortality rate of JDMS is less than 2%. JDMS is generally not associated with malignancy (in contrast to adult DM), and an occult malignancy work-up is not recommended.

Suggested Reading

Abdul-Aziz R, Yu C-Y, Adler B, et al. Muscle MRI at the time of questionable disease flares in Juvenile Dermatomyositis (JDM). Pediatr Rheumatol Online J. 2017;15:25. https://doi.org/10.1186/s12969-017-0154-4.

Enders FB, Bader-Meunier B, Baildam E, et al. Consensus-based recommendations for the management of juvenile dermatomyositis. Ann Rheum Dis. 2017;76:329–40.

Sun C, Lee J-H, Yang Y-H, et al. Juvenile dermatomyositis: a 20-year retrospective analysis of treatment and clinical outcomes. Pediatr Neonatal. 2015;56:31–9.

Part V
Reactions to External Causes

Chapter 17
Fixed Drug Eruption

Patricia Treadwell

17.1 Introduction

Fixed drug eruption (FDE) is a unique reaction to a variety of drugs. The drug reaction is categorized as a delayed-type hypersensitivity reaction mediated by CD8+ memory T cells [1].

17.2 Epidemiology

This particular drug eruption recurs in the same site(s) in response to exposure to the offending agent. The medications most often responsible are as follows: (1) non-steroidal anti-inflammatory drugs (NSAIDs), (2) other analgesics, (3) antibiotics, (4) laxatives, and (5) propranolol.

17.3 Clinical Findings

The lesions are typically oval or round with "dusky" (brownish or violaceous) centers (Fig. 17.1). On occasion, a bullae may form. They can occur anywhere on the body, including mucosal surfaces. Hyperpigmentation is a common feature; however, non-pigmented FDE (NPFDE) has been reported [2].

P. Treadwell (✉)
Department of Dermatology, Indiana University School of Medicine, Indianapolis, IN, USA
e-mail: ptreadwe@iupui.edu

© Springer Nature Switzerland AG 2021
P. Treadwell et al. (eds.), *Atlas of Adolescent Dermatology*,
https://doi.org/10.1007/978-3-030-58634-8_17

Fig. 17.1 FDE from
tetracycline

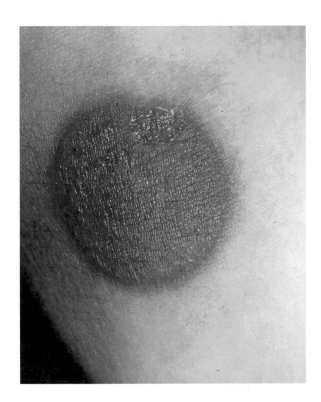

17.4 Laboratory

Histopathology shows a lichenoid infiltrate with necrotic keratinocytes and spongiosis. Drug challenge testing can be utilized to confirm the causative agent.

17.5 Treatment

Avoid the offending drug.

17.6 Prognosis

Avoidance of the drug trigger can minimize recurrences. Residual pigmentation can be noted in some cases.

References

1. Moya B, et al. Desquamating nonpigmenting fixed drug eruption with onycholysis due to amoxicillin in a child: cross-reactivity study. J Investig Allergol. 2020;30:149–51.
2. Streight KL, et al. A fixed drug eruption caused by mycophenolate. JAAD Case Rep. 2019;5:838–9.

Chapter 18
Phytophotodermatitis

Patricia Treadwell

18.1 Introduction

Phytophotodermatitis is a dermatitis that occurs following various furocoumarins coming in contact with the skin and subsequent ultraviolet exposure.

18.2 Epidemiology

Phytophotodermatitis can occur at any age. The furocoumarins associated with the dermatitis are found in citrus fruits (especially limes and lemons}, figs, wild dill and parsley, celery, fennel, and parsnip. The hyperpigmentation may be more evident in skin of color.

18.3 Clinical Findings

In milder cases, the cutaneous findings may consist of hyperpigmentation in an unusual pattern. In more severe cases, erythema and tense bullae may develop (Fig. 18.1). The tense bullae may be painful. Itching may be present.

P. Treadwell (✉)
Department of Dermatology, Indiana University School of Medicine, Indianapolis, IN, USA
e-mail: ptreadwe@iupui.edu

© Springer Nature Switzerland AG 2021
P. Treadwell et al. (eds.), *Atlas of Adolescent Dermatology*,
https://doi.org/10.1007/978-3-030-58634-8_18

Fig. 18.1 Phytophotodermatitis with erythematous
lesions, one with a bulla on
the back of the leg
after hiking

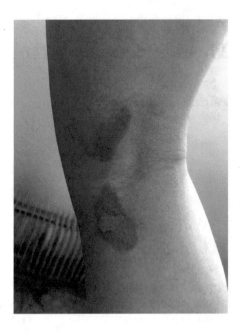

18.4   Laboratory

No laboratory testing is diagnostic nor necessary.

18.5   Treatment

If the lesions are symptomatic, topical corticosteroids or anti-pruritics can be prescribed.

18.6   Prognosis

The prognosis is generally good, since the hyperpigmentation will fade over time. Unfortunately, some cases have been misdiagnosed as child abuse based on the patterns of the lesions.

Avoiding the offending agents and ultraviolet exposure can minimize future occurrences.

Suggested Reading

Fitzpatrick JK, et al. Lime-induced Phytophotodermatitis. J Gen Intern Med. 2018;33:975.
Smith LG, et al. Phytophotodermatitis. Clin Pract Cases Emerg Med. 2017;1:146–7.

Part VI
Genodermatoses and Genetic Conditions

Chapter 19
Neurofibromatosis

Patricia Treadwell

19.1 Introduction

Neurocutaneous syndromes consist of neurologic issues in addition to cutaneous findings. One of the most common neurocutaneous disorders, which may be identified in the adolescent age group, is neurofibromatosis. Adolescents with neurofibromatosis are predisposed to both benign and malignant tumors.

19.2 Epidemiology

Neurofibromatosis 1 (NF1) occurs in approximately 1:2500–1:3000 individuals. NF1 occurs as a result of a germline mutation in one of the two alleles of the tumor suppressor gene NF1 on chromosome 17q11.2 (Ly KI et al). Neurofibromatosis 2 (NF2) is less common than NF1, occurring in 1:25,000 individuals. The mutation associated with NF2 occurs in neurofibromin-2 on chromosome 22q12. Patients with NF2 have acoustic neuromas – most typically bilateral. Inheritance of both NF1 and NF2 is considered to be autosomal dominant; however, the rate of spontaneous mutations is approximately 50% for both.

P. Treadwell (✉)
Department of Dermatology, Indiana University School of Medicine, Indianapolis, IN, USA
e-mail: ptreadwe@iupui.edu

© Springer Nature Switzerland AG 2021
P. Treadwell et al. (eds.), *Atlas of Adolescent Dermatology*,
https://doi.org/10.1007/978-3-030-58634-8_19

19.3   Clinical Findings

Cutaneous manifestations are significant in NF1. They represent the majority of the diagnostic criteria. The cutaneous findings with NF2 are less prominent. The most common cutaneous finding in NF1 is a café-au-lait macule (CALM) (Fig. 19.1). In skin of color, the café'-au-lait macules will be darker in color (Fig. 19.2). Other cutaneous findings, which are part of the diagnostic criteria, are neurofibromas, freckling of skin folds (Fig. 19.3), Lisch nodules, and plexiform neuromas. Plexiform neuromas have an increased risk of transformation into a malignant peripheral nerve sheath tumor (MPNST).

Other tumors noted are rhabdomyosarcomas.

Other associated findings with NF1 are pruritus, macrocephaly, learning disabilities, and skeletal abnormalities (short stature, osteopenia, scoliosis, and sphenoid wing dysplasia).

As mentioned above, NF2 has less prominent cutaneous findings when compared to NF1. Associated findings with NF2 are meningiomas of the brain, and schwannomas of the dorsal roots of the spinal cord.

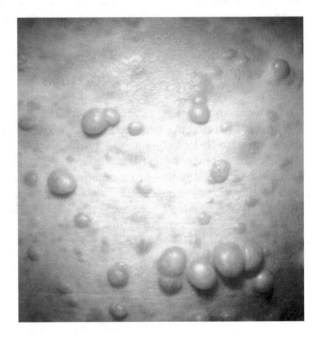

Fig. 19.1 Multiple neurofibromas with a CALM in the upper part of the photograph in a patient with NF1

Fig. 19.2 CALM which is a more brown in skin of color

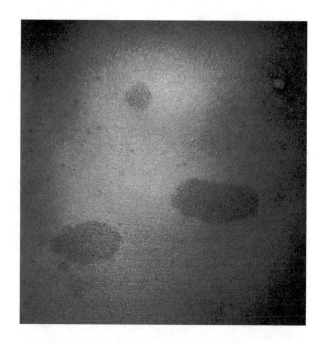

Fig. 19.3 Axillary freckling in a patient with NF1

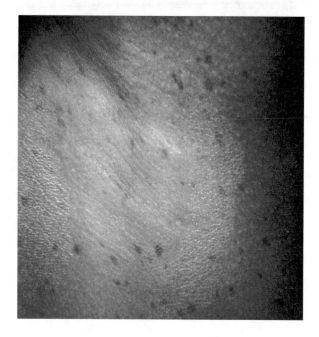

19.4 Laboratory

Genetic testing may be indicated when the diagnostic criteria are not confirmatory or mosaicism is suspected. Tumor surveillance is an ongoing issue. Radiation therapy is to be avoided in NF1 patients due to the increased risk of developing radiation-induced malignancies [1].

19.5 Treatment

In light of the predisposition for tumors, health supervision includes tumor surveillance especially if specific findings are noted. Tumor-specific treatment may include surgical excision and/or chemotherapy. As noted above, radiation therapy is used with caution [2].

19.6 Prognosis

Life expectancy is shortened due to malignancy and has been estimated between 54 and 71.5 years [3].

References

1. Kersak JL, et al. Neurofibromatosis: a review of NF1, NF2, and schwannomatosis. J Pediatr Genet. 2016;5:98–104.
2. Ly KI, et al. The diagnosis and management of neurofibromatosis type 1. Med Clin N Am. 2019;103:1035–54.
3. Wilding A, et al. Life expectancy in hereditary cancer predisposing diseases: an observational study. J Med Genet. 2012;49:264–9.

Chapter 20
Tuberous Sclerosis Complex

Patricia Treadwell

20.1 Introduction

Tuberous sclerosis complex (TSC) is a neurocutaneous disorder characterized by mutations in the TSC1 gene (encoding of hamartin) or TSC2 gene (encoding of tuberin). The mutations result in dysregulation of cellular hyperplasia.

20.2 Epidemiology

TSC occurs at a rate of 1:6000 to 1:10,000 live births [1]. TSC1 is located on chromosome 9q34 and encodes hamartin. TSC2 is located on chromosome 16p13 and encodes tuberin. Inheritance of TSC is considered to be autosomal dominant; however, the rate of spontaneous mutations is approximately 70%.

20.3 Clinical Findings

Cutaneous findings include hypomelanotic macules (ash leaf spots), facial angiofibromas (Fig. 20.1), periungual fibromas (Fig. 20.2), and connective tissue nevi – fibrous cephalic plaque (on the head and neck) (Fig. 20.3), or shagreen patch (often located on the lower back.

Other associated findings are epilepsy, learning difficulties, autism, and attention deficit disorders.

P. Treadwell (✉)
Department of Dermatology, Indiana University School of Medicine, Indianapolis, IN, USA
e-mail: ptreadwe@iupui.edu

© Springer Nature Switzerland AG 2021
P. Treadwell et al. (eds.), *Atlas of Adolescent Dermatology*,
https://doi.org/10.1007/978-3-030-58634-8_20

Fig. 20.1 Facial
angiofibromas

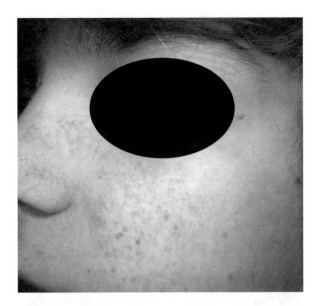

Fig. 20.2 Periungual
fibroma

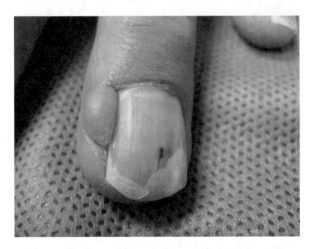

Hamartomas which may develop are retinal hamartomas, subependymal giant cell tumors (SGCTs), cardiac rhabdomyomas, renal and non-renal angiomyolipomas (AMLs), and pulmonary lymphangiomyomatosis (LAM).

Dental enamel pits and intraoral fibromas may be noted.

20.4 Laboratory

Imaging may show "cortical tubers" (occurring in about 80% of TSC patients), which are composed of abnormal neurons and glia.

Fig. 20.3 Fibrous
cephalic plaque

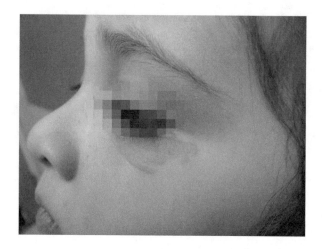

20.5   Treatment

Specific guidelines for surveillance assist in management of the hamartomas and associated findings. Consultation with neurology can be helpful to treat epilepsy. Topical or systemic mTOR inhibitors have been useful for specific complications.

20.6   Prognosis

Although the hamartomas are typically benign, they may cause a mass effect.

Reference

1. Randle SC. Tuberous sclerosis complex: a review. Pediatr Ann. 2017;46:e166–71.

Chapter 21
Erythropoietic Protoporphyria

Julie Prendiville

21.1   Introduction

Erythropoietic protoporphyria (EPP) is a rare genetic disorder of heme biosynthesis characterized clinically by acute pain on sun exposure.

21.2   Epidemiology

EPP is the most common porphyria of childhood. It may present or be first diagnosed in adolescence.

Inheritance is autosomal recessive. It is caused by a combination of loss of function mutations and low expression allelic variants in the *FECH* gene. Deficiency of the enzyme ferrochelatase leads to accumulation of protoporphyrin IX in circulating erythrocytes. Following exposure to sunlight, these protoporphyrins cause acute cutaneous phototoxicity. Accumulation of protoporphyrins in the liver may result in hepatotoxicity and cholestasis.

X-linked protoporphyria, caused by mutations in *ALAS2,* has a similar clinical presentation to EPP.

J. Prendiville (✉)
Department of Pediatrics, University of British Columbia, Vancouver, BC, Canada
e-mail: jprendiville@sidra.org

© Springer Nature Switzerland AG 2021
P. Treadwell et al. (eds.), *Atlas of Adolescent Dermatology*,
https://doi.org/10.1007/978-3-030-58634-8_21

21.3   Clinical Findings

Symptoms occur shortly after sun exposure, most commonly on the face, dorsal hands, arms, and feet. Objective clinical findings are often absent despite excruciating pain. Variable erythema and edema may be observed (Fig. 21.1). Erosions and crusting of the skin are uncommon. Chronic atrophic changes on the face or dorsal hands may result from severe phototoxic reactions or recurrent sun exposure.

21.4   Laboratory

Laboratory investigation shows elevated levels of free erythrocyte protoporphyrin. The diagnosis may be confirmed by sequencing of the *FECH* (or *ALAS2*) gene. Patients require monitoring for liver dysfunction, anemia, and vitamin D deficiency.

Fig. 21.1 Erythema of dorsal hands in EPP

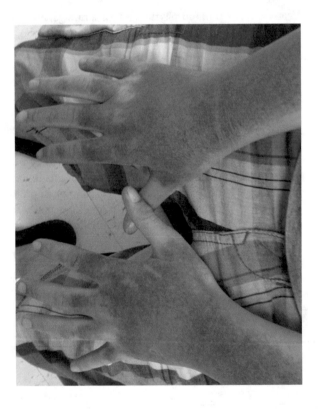

21.5 Treatment

Sun avoidance is the mainstay of treatment. A UV meter may be helpful to indicate the times and months when protective clothing, hats, gloves, umbrellas, and tinted windows are required. Topical sunscreens are of limited benefit. Oral betacarotene and alfamelanotide have been reported to improve sun tolerance.

21.6 Prognosis

Social isolation and lifestyle changes may significantly impair quality of life. A small subset of patients have severe progressive liver disease.

Suggested Reading

Balwani M. Erythropoietic protoporphyria and X-linked protoporphyria: pathophysiology, genetics, clinical manifestations, and management. Mol Gen Metabol. 2019;128:298.
Juengling A-M, Boulter EL, Kava MP. Erythropoietic protoporphyria: a rare cause of painful hands and feet. J Paediatr Child Health. 2019;55:236–8.

Chapter 22
Nevus Sebaceous

Julie Prendiville

22.1 Introduction

The nevus sebaceous is a congenital hamartoma of epidermal structures including hair follicles and sebaceous and apocrine glands. It is commonly located on the scalp or face. The appearance of a nevus sebaceous changes after puberty, and this can present as a concern in adolescence.

22.2 Epidemiology

An isolated nevus sebaceous occurs in approximately 0.3% of newborns. It is caused by a postzygotic somatic *HRAS,* or less commonly *KRAS*, gene variant. Nevus sebaceous may be associated with other congenital developmental anomalies, as in the rare Schimmelpenning syndrome.

22.3 Clinical Findings

The typical nevus sebaceous is a yellow-orange plaque with a pebbly or velvety surface located on the scalp or face (Fig. 22.1). It varies in size from one to several centimeters and can be round, oval, or linear in shape. Lesions on the scalp present

J. Prendiville (✉)
Department of Pediatrics, University of British Columbia, Vancouver, BC, Canada
e-mail: jprendiville@sidra.org

© Springer Nature Switzerland AG 2021
P. Treadwell et al. (eds.), *Atlas of Adolescent Dermatology*,
https://doi.org/10.1007/978-3-030-58634-8_22

Fig. 22.1 Nevus sebaceous of the left temple area

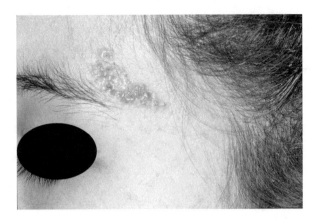

as a congenital area of circumscribed alopecia. A thickened or verrucous appearance may develop in adolescence when the sebaceous and apocrine glands enlarge with puberty.

22.4 Laboratory

Histopathology following excision (or biopsy) shows immature hair follicles, numerous hyperplastic sebaceous and apocrine glands, and overlying epidermal hyperplasia.

22.5 Treatment

Treatment is by surgical excision. Continued observation is also an acceptable option with sun protection.

22.6 Prognosis

Secondary tumors may develop within a nevus sebaceous in adolescence or adult life. These are usually benign but malignant tumors can occur.

Suggested Reading

Aslam A, Salam A, Griffiths CEM, McGrath JA. Naevus sebaceus: a mosaic RASopathy. Clin Exp Dermatol. 2014;39:1–6.

Chapter 23
Nevus of Ota and Ito

Patricia Treadwell

23.1 Introduction

Nevus of Ota (nevus fuscoceruleus ophthalmomaxillaris) and Ito (nevus fuscoceruleus acromiodeltoideus) are lesions that are examples of dermal melanocytosis.
Dermal melanocytosis results from abnormal migration of neural crest cells with
subsequent pigmentary changes from the ectopic melanocytes in the dermis.

23.2 Epidemiology

Nevus of Ota and Ito are more common in patients with African or Asian ancestry
although they can occur in all races. Females are affected more often than males [1].
There are two peaks of presentation, one at birth, with a second peak near puberty.
A few cases of later onset have been reported in the literature [2].

23.3 Clinical Findings

The distribution of pigment in the nevus of Ota typically corresponds to the ophthal-
mic and maxillary branches of the trigeminal nerve, less commonly corresponding
to the mandibular branch. Two-thirds of patients will have ocular pigmentation
(oculodermal melanocytosis) (Fig. 23.1). In nevus of Ito, the distribution involves

P. Treadwell (✉)
Department of Dermatology, Indiana University School of Medicine, Indianapolis, IN, USA
e-mail: ptreadwe@iupui.edu

© Springer Nature Switzerland AG 2021
P. Treadwell et al. (eds.), *Atlas of Adolescent Dermatology*,
https://doi.org/10.1007/978-3-030-58634-8_23

Fig. 23.1 Patient with
nevus of Ota. Also has
ocular pigmentation

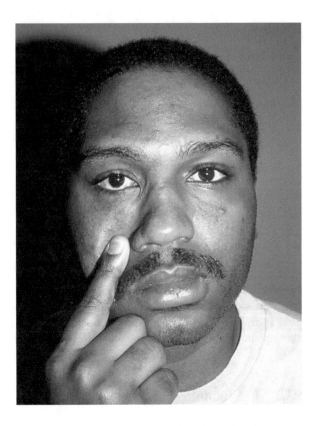

posterior supraclavicular area and lateral neck. In both entities, dermal melanocytosis is responsible for the clinical appearance, with distribution being the main difference between them.

23.4   Laboratory

Histopathology shows pigmented dendritic melanocytes dissecting dermal collagen bundles in the dermis.

23.5   Treatment

A variety of lasers have been used to treat nevus of Ota and Ito [3]. Because of the increased risk of glaucoma in eyes with oculodermal melanocytosis, routine ophthalmologic exams are recommended [3].

23.6   Prognosis

Adolescents without complications such as glaucoma have a good prognosis. Malignant melanoma occurring in the skin, meninges, and/or eye associated with these lesions is quite rare.

References

1. Kumar MA. Nevus of Ota associated with nevus of Ito. Indian J Dermatol Venereol Leprol. 2004;70:112–3.
2. Khurana A, Gupta A, Sardana K, et al. Late-onset naevus of Ota: a case series of six patients. Clin Exp Dermatol. 2018;44:703. https://doi.org/10.1111/ced.13839.
3. Shah VV, Bray FN, Aldahan AS, et al. Lasers and nevus of Ota: a comprehensive review. Lasers Med Sci. 2016;31:179–85.

Part VII
Tumors and Nodular Lesions Nodular

Chapter 24
Pilomatrixoma

Patricia Treadwell

24.1 Introduction

Pilomatrixoma is a benign adnexal tumor. It is also known as a calcifying epithelioma of Malherbe. It consists of benign hyperplasia of the hair follicle matrix cells.

24.2 Epidemiology

Pilomatrixomas may occur at any age; nonetheless, they most often are noted prior to age 20. Generally, these lesions do not have a known genetic predisposition; however, multiple lesions have been associated with myotonic dystrophy, Gardner syndrome, Rubenstein-Taybi syndrome, and trisomy 9 (among others). Some recent studies have identified an association with mutations in Wnt (wingless and Int-1) signaling pathways [1].

24.3 Clinical Findings

Pilomatrixomas are typically solitary nodule and noted most often on the face or proximal extremities. The lesions tend to be slow growing, firm lesions with an irregular surface (Fig. 24.1). Some of the lesions will have a violaceous discoloration initially. Pilomatrixomas may develop calcium deposits and become very hard.

P. Treadwell (✉)
Department of Dermatology, Indiana University School of Medicine, Indianapolis, IN, USA
e-mail: ptreadwe@iupui.edu

© Springer Nature Switzerland AG 2021
P. Treadwell et al. (eds.), *Atlas of Adolescent Dermatology*,
https://doi.org/10.1007/978-3-030-58634-8_24

Fig. 24.1 Irregular surface
of this pilomatrixoma
below the medial eyebrow

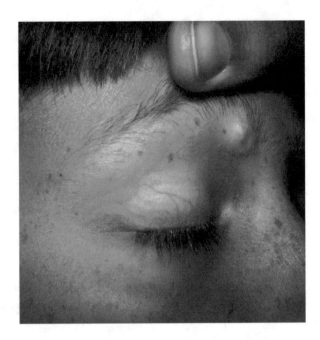

24.4   Laboratory

When a biopsy is performed, the findings are proliferation of basaloid cells, shadow
cells, or both [1].

24.5   Treatment

The lesions will sometimes resolve spontaneously over a period of several months.
If they become repeatedly flared or superinfected, they can be surgically excised.

24.6   Prognosis

When the lesions resolve spontaneously, minimal scarring is noted. When they are
surgically excised, a healed surgical scar will result.

Reference

1. Jones CD, et al. Pilomatrixoma: a comprehensive review of the literature. Am J Dermatopathol.
   2018;40:631–41.

Chapter 25
Epidermal Inclusion Cyst

Patricia Treadwell

25.1 Introduction

Epidermal inclusion cysts (EICs) (aka epidermoid cysts) are cystic lesions with an epithelial lining, which can develop in adolescence and early adulthood. Some may develop following the inflammatory phase of nodular acne lesions.

25.2 Epidemiology

In particular, EICs following acne lesions may be noted on the upper back, chest, neck, and face. They also can be seen anywhere on the body. Most often the lesions are solitary when not associated with a genetic syndrome.

25.3 Clinical Findings

An EIC is a slow growing cystic lesion with components above and below the surface of the skin. Some lesions may have central punctum, which was previously a follicular opening (Fig. 25.1).

P. Treadwell (✉)

Department of Dermatology, Indiana University School of Medicine, Indianapolis, IN, USA

e-mail: ptreadwe@iupui.edu

© Springer Nature Switzerland AG 2021

P. Treadwell et al. (eds.), *Atlas of Adolescent Dermatology*,

https://doi.org/10.1007/978-3-030-58634-8_25

Fig. 25.1 Greater than 5
EICs in addition to 3
scarred areas from I&D on
the back of a patient
with acne

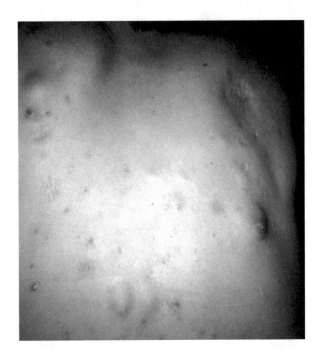

25.4 Laboratory

The material expressed from an EIC has been described as "cheesy." The contents
of the EICs are generally sterile if cultured. A biopsy will show a distended infun-
dibulum with an epithelial lining, which resembles the epidermis with a granular
layer and keratin lamellae [1].

25.5 Treatment

Treatment of asymptomatic lesions may not be necessary. The lesions tend to be
slow growing; however, they can exhibit inflammation or develop a secondary bacterial infection. Incision and drainage (I&D) tends not to be an effective treatment
especially if a portion of the lining is still present. Complete surgical excision of the
cyst with its lining can result in complete resolution.

25.6 Prognosis

The untreated lesions tend to be persistent but may become a cosmetic issue. Scarring may result from I&D or surgical excision.

Reference

1. Hoang VT, et al. Overview of epidermoid cyst. Eur J Radiol Open. 2019;6:291–301.

Chapter 26
Pyogenic Granuloma

Patricia Treadwell

26.1 Introduction

The term "pyogenic granuloma" is unfortunately somewhat of a misnomer. The lesion is not typically pyogenic nor is it a granuloma. The lesion has also been labeled a lobular capillary hemangioma – an acquired vascular lesion.

26.2 Epidemiology

Pyogenic granulomas are most often noted in childhood and adolescence. The etiology is theorized to be neovascularization. This can occur following trauma or can also be seen arising within a nevus flammeus [1].

26.3 Clinical Findings

The lesion usually is a reddish to violaceous lobulated nodule (Fig. 26.1). The surface may become eroded. In some cases, it can become pedunculated (Fig. 26.2). The history given by the patient and/or caregivers is that it often spontaneously bleeds. They are most often located on the fingers, face, and oral mucosa.

P. Treadwell (✉)
Department of Dermatology, Indiana University School of Medicine, Indianapolis, IN, USA
e-mail: ptreadwe@iupui.edu

© Springer Nature Switzerland AG 2021
P. Treadwell et al. (eds.), *Atlas of Adolescent Dermatology*,
https://doi.org/10.1007/978-3-030-58634-8_26

Fig. 26.1 Lobulated
pyogenic granuloma

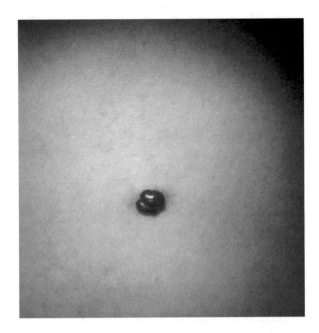

Fig. 26.2 Pedunculated
pyogenic granuloma

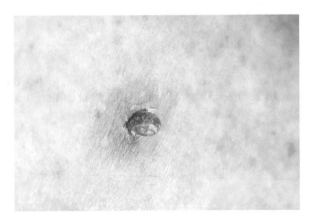

26.4   Laboratory

Histopathology shows a proliferation of capillaries and fibroplasia.

26.5   Treatment

Surgical excision with curettage and/or cautery was previously considered the best
option; however, recently, topical beta blockers have been noted to be useful [2].

26.6 Prognosis

Incomplete excision may result in recurrence.

References

1. Shruti S, Fouzia S, Vasanthi R, Ramesh V. Recurrent pyogenic granuloma over nevus flammeus. Indian J Dermatol Venereol Leprol. 2019;85:236.
2. Goetze AC, Mayumi Kubo Sasaya E, Bochnia Cerci F, Tolkachjov SN, Werner B. Pyogenic granuloma of the lip with complete resolution after topical propranolol. J Drugs Dermatol. 2019;18:1061–2.

Part VIII
Lymphocytic Disorders

Chapter 27
Pityriasis Lichenoides et Varioliformis Acuta

Julie Prendiville

27.1 Introduction

Pityriasis lichenoides is an inflammatory skin disorder of unknown etiology. There are two variants with overlapping features: (1) pityriasis lichenoides chronica (PLC) and (2) pityriasis lichenoides et varioliformis acuta (PLEVA). Febrile ulceronecrotic Mucha-Haberman disease is a severe form of PLEVA with systemic manifestations.

27.2 Epidemiology

The exact prevalence is unknown. Pityriasis lichenoides predominantly affects children and young adults, including adolescents.

27.3 Clinical Findings

Widespread erythematous papules with overlying adherent scale are characteristic (Figs. 27.1 and 27.2). PLEVA papules show central hemorrhagic ulceration and crusting and may be mistaken for varicella infection or insect bites. White, or pigmented, macules are seen where previous lesions have resolved. Symptoms are variable and may be absent. The rare febrile ulceronecrotic Mucha-Haberman disease is characterized by large, painful ulcerating lesions associated with high fever and signs and symptoms of multisystem inflammatory disease.

J. Prendiville (✉)
Department of Pediatrics, University of British Columbia, Vancouver, BC, Canada
e-mail: jprendiville@sidra.org

© Springer Nature Switzerland AG 2021
P. Treadwell et al. (eds.), *Atlas of Adolescent Dermatology*,
https://doi.org/10.1007/978-3-030-58634-8_27

115

Fig. 27.1 PLEVA lesions of the lateral foot

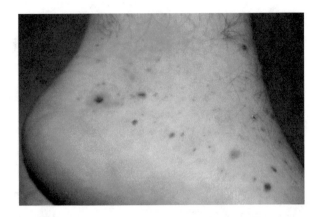

Fig. 27.2 PLEVA lesions of the ankle showing petechiae and scale

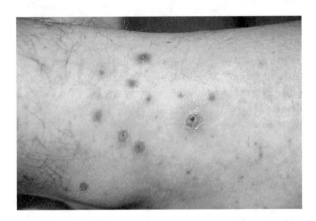

27.4 Laboratory

The diagnosis is established by skin biopsy. Laboratory markers of inflammation are elevated in febrile ulceronecrotic Mucha-Haberman disease.

27.5 Treatment

Prolonged courses of an oral antibiotic (erythromycin or tetracycline) or narrow-band UVB phototherapy are the most commonly prescribed treatments. Systemic anti-inflammatory drugs are reserved for cases of recalcitrant or severe disease.

27.6 Prognosis

The course is usually benign and self-limiting with a waxing and waning course over several months or years. Post inflammatory hypopigmented macules are common in both variants. Ulcerating lesions result in atrophic scarring. There are rare instances of PLC progressing to mycosis fungoides, a type of cutaneous T-cell lymphoma.

Suggested Reading

Bowers S, Warshaw EM. Pityriasis lichenoides and its subtypes. J Am Acad Dermatol. 2006;55:557–72.
Geller L, Antonov NK, Lauren CT, et al. Pityriasis lichenoides in childhood: review of clinical presentation and treatment options. Pediatr Dermatol. 2015;32:579–92.

Chapter 28
Pigmented Purpuric Dermatosis

Julie Prendiville

28.1 Introduction

Pigmented purpura refers to a group of benign skin disorders characterized by patches of purpura and petechiae with pigmentation resulting from hemosiderin deposition. The lower extremities are primarily involved. The appearance can be a cosmetic concern for adolescents.

28.2 Epidemiology

Pigmented purpura is relatively uncommon. It is seen in all age groups. The cause is unknown.

28.3 Clinical Findings

At least five different subtypes are described but there may be overlap between these disorders. The subtypes are as follows: (1) Schamberg disease (progressive pigmentary purpura), (2) Majocchi disease (purpura annularis telangiectoides), (3) Lichen aureus, (4) Gougerot-Blum purpura, and (5) eczematoid-like purpura (eczematoid-like purpura of Doucas and Kapetanakis).

Schamberg disease (progressive pigmentary purpura) is the most common variant in children and adolescents. It presents with non-palpable reddish-brown areas

J. Prendiville (✉)
Department of Pediatrics, University of British Columbia, Vancouver, BC, Canada
e-mail: jprendiville@sidra.org

© Springer Nature Switzerland AG 2021
P. Treadwell et al. (eds.), *Atlas of Adolescent Dermatology*,
https://doi.org/10.1007/978-3-030-58634-8_28

of purpura and pigmentation, within which punctate petechiae ("cayenne pepper spots") are visible (Fig. 28.1).

Majocchi disease (purpura annularis telangiectoides) occurs in adolescent patients and is characterized by petechiae, purpura, and telangiectases in an annular pattern (Fig. 28.2).

Lichen aureus is a subtype of pigmented purpura with few and localized lesions. The pigmentation typically has an orange-yellow hue.

Less common variants have a lichenoid morphology or overlying scale and may be associated with pruritus. Rarely, mycosis fungoides can present with or mimic a pigmented purpuric dermatosis.

Pigmented purpura primarily affects the lower extremities. It occasionally affects the upper limbs and may rarely be generalized. It is usually asymptomatic.

28.4 Laboratory

Histopathology typically shows a perivascular lymphocytic infiltrate with extravasation of red blood cells and hemosiderin deposition in the dermis.

The platelet count and coagulation studies are normal. Laboratory markers of inflammation are not elevated.

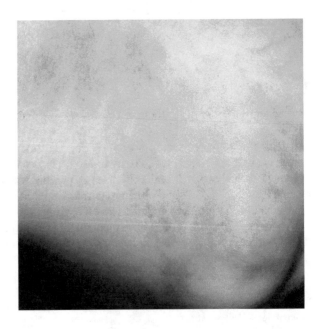

Fig. 28.1 Schamberg disease with reddish-brown areas with petechiae

Fig. 28.2 Purpura
annularis telangiectoides

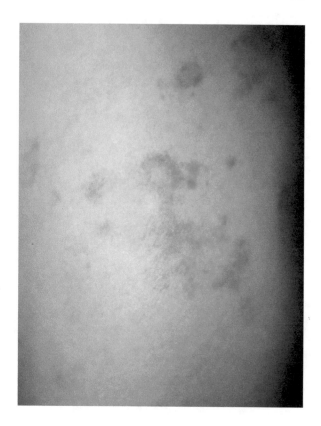

28.5   Treatment

Treatment is challenging and not necessary for asymptomatic patients unless there is concern about cosmesis. Topical steroids and calcineurin inhibitors are often prescribed. Narrow-band UVB phototherapy can be helpful in some cases.

28.6   Prognosis

The course is variable. Lesions may persist or recur from several months to many years.

Suggested Reading

Coulombe J, Jean S-E, Hatami A, et al. Pigmented purpuric dermatosis: clinicopathologic characterization in a pediatric series. Pediatr Dermatol. 2015;32:358–62.
Kim DH, Seo SH, Ahn HH, et al. Characteristics and clinical manifestations of pigmented purpuric dermatosis. Ann Dermatol. 2015;27:404–10.

Index

© Springer Nature Switzerland AG 2021
P. Treadwell et al. (eds.), *Atlas of Adolescent Dermatology*,
https://doi.org/10.1007/978-3-030-58634-8